# Discourses on a Sober and Temperate Life

## By Lewis Cornaro

The author of the following discourses, Lewis Cornaro, was descended from one of the most illustrious families in Venice, but by the ill conduct of some of his relations, had the misfortune to be deprived of the dignity of a nobleman, and excluded from all honours and public employments in the state. Chagrined at this unmerited disgrace, he retired to Padua, and married a lady of the family of Spiltemberg, whose name was Veronica. Being in possession of a good estate, he was very desirous of having children; and after a long expectation of this happiness, his wife was delivered of a daughter, to whom he gave the name of Clara. This was his only child, who afterwards was married to John, the son of Fantini Cornaro, of a rich family in Cyprus, while that island belonged to the republic of Venice. Though he was far advanced in life when his daughter Clara came into the world, yet he lived to see her very old, and the mother of eight sons and three daughters. He was a man of sound understanding, determined courage and resolution. In his younger days, he had contracted infirmities by intemperance, and by indulging his too great propensity to anger; but when he perceived the ill consequence of his irregularities, he had command enough of himself to subdue his passion and inordinate appetites. By means of great sobriety, and a strict regimen in his diet, he recovered his health and vigour, which he preserved to an extreme old age. At a very advanced stage of life he wrote the following discourses, wherein he acquaints us with the irregularity of his youth, his reformation of manners, and the hopes he entertained of living a long time. Nor was he mistaken in his expectation, for he resigned his last breath without any agony, sitting in an elbow chair, being above an hundred years old. This happened at Padua, the 26th of April, 1566. His lady, almost as old as himself, survived him but a short time, and died an early death. They were both interred in St. Anthony's church, without pomp, pursuant to their testamentary directions.

These discourses, though written in Cornaro's old age, were penned at different times, and published separately: The first, which he wrote at the age of eighty-three, is intitled, A Treatise on a Sober Life, in which he declares war against every kind of intemperance; and his vigorous old age speaks in favour of his precepts. The second treatise he composed at the age of eighty-six: it contains farther encomiums on sobriety, and points out the means of mending a bad constitution. He says, that he came into the world with a choleric disposition, but that his temperate way of life had enabled him to subdue it. The third, which he wrote at the age of ninety-one, is intitled, An Earnest Exhortation to a Sober Life; here he uses the strongest arguments to persuade mankind to embrace a temperate life, as the means of attaining a healthy and vigorous old age. The fourth and last, is a letter to Barbaro, Patriarch of Aquileia, written at the age of ninety-five; it contains a lively description of the healthy, vigour, and perfect use of all his faculties, which he had the happiness of enjoying at that advanced period of life.

This useful work was translated some years ago into English, under the title of Sure and certain methods of attaining a long and healthy life. The translator seems rather to have made use of a French version than of the Italian original; he has likewise omitted several passages of the Italian, and the whole is rather a paraphrase than a translation. This has induced us to give the public an exact and faithful version of that excellent performance, from the Venice edition in 8vo, in the year 1620 [1]: and as a proof of the merit and authenticity of the work, we beg leave to quote Mr. Addison's recommendation of it, SPECTATOR, Vol. iii, No 195.

"The most remarkable instance of the efficacy of temperance, towards the procuring long life, is what we meet with in a little book published by Lewis Cornaro, the Venetian; which I rather mention, because it is of undoubted credit, as the late Venetian ambassador, who was of the same family, attested more than once in conversation, when he resided in England. Cornaro, who was the author of the little treatise I am mentioning, was of an infirm constitution, till about forty, when, by obstinately persisting in an exact course of temperance, he recovered a perfect state of health; insomuch that at fourscore he published his book, which has been translated into English under the title of, Sure and certain methods of attaining a long and healthy life. He lived to give a third or fourth edition of it, and after having passed his hundredth year, died without pain or agony, and like one who falls asleep.

The treatise I mention has been taken notice of by several eminent authors, and is written with such spirit of chearfulness, religion, and good sense, as are the natural concomitants of temperance and sobriety. The mixture of the old man in it, is rather a recommendation than a discredit to it."

[1] The first edition was published by the author at Padua, in 4to, A.D. 1558.

A TREATISE ON A SOBER LIFE

It is a thing past all doubt, that custom, by time, becomes a second nature, forcing men to use that, whether good or bad, to which they have been habituated: nay, we see habit, in many things, get the better of reason. This is so undeniably true, that virtuous men, by conversing with the wicked, very often fall into the same vicious course of life. The contrary, likewise, we see sometimes happen; viz. that, as good morals easily change to bad, so bad morals change again to good. For instance: let a wicked man, who was once virtuous, keep company with a virtuous man, and he will again become virtuous; and this alteration can be attributed to nothing but the force of habit, which is, indeed, very great. Seeing many examples of this; and besides, considering that, in consequence of this great force of habit, three bad customs have got footing in Italy within a few years, even within my own memory; the first flattery and ceremoniousness: the second Lutheranism [2], which some have most preposterously embraced; the third intemperance; and that these three vices, like so many cruel monsters, leagued, as indeed they are, against mankind, have gradually prevailed so far, as to rob civil life of its sincerity, the soul of its piety, and the body of its health; I have resolved to treat of the last of these vices, and prove that it is an abuse, in order to extirpate it, if possible. As to the second, Lutheranism, and the first, flattery, I am certain, that some great genius or another will soon undertake the task of exposing their deformity, and effectually suppressing them. Therefore, I firmly hope, that, before I die, I shall see these three abuses conquered and driven out of Italy; and this country of course restored to its former laudable and virtuous customs.

[2] The author writes with the prejudice of a zealous Roman Catholic against the doctrine of the Reformation, which he here distinguishes by the name of Lutheranism. This was owing to the artifices of the Romish clergy in those days, by whom the reformed religion was misinterpreted, as introductive of licentiousness and debauchery.

To come then to that abuse, of which I am proposed to speak, namely, intemperance; I say, that it is a great pity it should have prevailed so much, as entirely to banish sobriety. Though all are agreed, that intemperance is the offspring of gluttony, and sober living of abstemiousness; the former, nevertheless, is considered a virtue and a mark of distinction, and the latter, as dishonourable and the badge of avarice. Such mistaken notions are entirely owing to the power of custom, established by our senses and irregular appetites; these have blinded and besotted men to such a degree, that, leaving the paths of virtue, they have followed those of vice, which lead them before their time to an old age, burthened with strange and mortal infirmities, so as to render them quite decrepid before forty, contrary to the effects of sobriety, which, before it was banished by this destructive intemperance, used to keep men sound and hearty to the age of eighty and upwards. O wretched and unhappy Italy! do you not see, that intemperance murders every year more of your subjects, than you could lose by the most cruel plague, or by fire and sword in many battles? Those truly shameful feasts, no so much in fashion, and so intolerably profuse, that no tables are large enough to hold the dishes, which renders it necessary to heap them one upon another; those feasts, I say, are so many battles; and how is it possible to support nature by such a variety of contrary and unwholesome foods? Put a stop to this abuse, for God's sake, for there is not, I am certain of it, a vice more abominable than this in the eyes of the Divine Majesty. Drive away this new kind of death, and you have banished the plague, which, though it formerly used to make such havock, now does little or no mischief, owing to the laudable practice of attending more to the goodness of the provisions brought to our markets. There are means still left to banish intemperance, and such means too, that every man may have recourse to them without any assistance. Nothing more is requisite for this purpose, than to live up to the simplicity dictated by nature, which teaches us to be content with little, to pursue the medium of holy abstemiousness and divine reason, and to accustom ourselves to eat no more than is absolutely necessary to support life; considering, that what exceeds this, is disease and death, and merely gives the palate satisfaction, which, though but momentary, brings on the body a long and lasting train of disagreeable sensations and diseases, and at length destroys it along with the soul. How many friends of mine, men of the finest understanding and most amiable disposition, have I seen carried off by this plague in the flower of their youth? who, where they now living, would be an ornament to the public, whose company I should enjoy with as much pleasure, as I now feel concern at their loss.

In order, therefore, to put a stop to so great an evil, I have resolved by this short discourse to demonstrate, that intemperance is an abuse which may be easily removed, and that the good old sober living may be substituted in its stead; and this I undertake more readily, as many young men of the best understanding, knowing that it is a vice, have requested it of me, moved thereto by seeing their fathers drop off in the flower of their youth, and me so sound and hearty at the age of eighty-one. They expressed a desire to reach the same term, nature not forbidding us to wish for longevity; and old-age being, in fact, that time of life in which prudence can be best exercised, and the fruits of all the other virtues enjoyed with less opposition, the passions being then so subdued, that man gives himself up entirely to reason. They beseeched me to let them know the method pursued by me to attain it; and then finding them intent on so laudable a pursuit, I have resolved to treat of that method, in order to be of service not only to them, but to all those who may be willing to peruse this discourse. I shall, therefore, give my reasons for renouncing intemperance, and betaking myself to a sober course of life; declare freely the method pursued by me for that purpose; and then set forth the effects of so good an habit upon me; whence it may be clearly gathered, how easy it is to remove the abuse of intemperance. I shall conclude, by shewing how many conveniencies and blessings are the consequences of a sober life.

I say then, that the heavy train of infirmities, which had not only invaded, but even made great inroads in my constitution, were my motives for renouncing intemperance, to which I had been greatly addicted; so that, in consequence of it, and the badness of my constitution, my stomach being exceedingly cold and moist, I was fallen into different kinds of disorders, such as pains in my stomach, and often stitches, and spices of the gout; attended by, what was still worse, an almost continual slow fever, a stomach generally out of order, and a perpetual thirst. From these natural and acquired disorders the best delivery I had to hope for, was death, to put an end to the pains and miseries of life; a period very remote in the regular course of nature, though I had hastened it by my irregular manner of living. Finding myself, therefore, in such unhappy circumstances between my thirty-fifth and fortieth year, every thing that could be thought of having been tried to no purpose to relieve me, the physicians gave me to understand, that there was but one method left to get the better of my complaints, provided I would resolve to use it, and patiently persevere in it. This was a sober and regular life, which the assured me would be still of the greatest service to me, and would be as powerful in its effects, as the intemperance and irregular one had been, in reducing me to the present low condition: and that I might be fully satisfied of its salutary effects, for though by my irregularities I was become infirm, I was not reduced so low, but that a temperate life, the opposite in every respect to an intemperate one, might still entirely recover me. And besides, it in fact appears, such a regular life, whilst observed, preserves men of a bad constitution, and far gone in years, just as a contrary course has the power to destroy those of the best constitution, and in their prime; for this plain reason, that different modes of life are attended by different effects; art following, even herein, the steps of nature, with equal power to correct natural vices and imperfections. This is obvious in husbandry and the like. They added, that if I did not immediately have recourse to such a regimen, I could receive no benefit from it in a few months, and that in a few more I must resign myself to death.

These solid and convincing arguments made such an impression on me, that, mortified as I was besides, by the thoughts of dying in the prime of life, and at the same time perpetually tormented by various diseases, I immediately concluded, that the foregoing contrary effects could not be produced but by contrary modes of living; and, therefore, full of hopes, resolved, in order to avoid at once both death and disease, to betake myself to a regular course of life. Having, upon this, enquired of them what rules I should follow, they told me, that I must not use any food, solid or liquid, but such as, being generally prescribed to sick persons, is, for that reason, called diet, and both very sparingly. These directions, to say the truth, they had before given me; but it was at a time of life when, impatient of such restraint, and finding myself satiated, as it were, with such food, I could not put up with it, and therefore eat freely of every thing I liked best; and likewise, feeling myself in a manner parched up by the heat of my disease, made no scruple of drinking, and in large quantities, the wines that best pleased my palate. This indeed, like all other patients, I kept a secret from my physicians. But, when I had once resolved to live sparingly, and according to the dictates of reason, seeing that is was no difficult matter, nay, that it was my duty as a man so to do, I entered with so much resolution upon this new course of life, that nothing has been since able to divert me from it. The consequence was, that in a few days I began to perceive, that such a course agreed with me very well; and by pursuing it, in less than a year, I found myself (some persons, perhaps, will not believe it) entirely freed from all my complaints.

Having thus recovered my health, I began seriously to consider the power of temperance, and say to myself, that if this virtue had efficacy enough to subdue such grievous disorders as mine, it must have still greater to preserve me in health, to help my bad constitution, and comfort my very weak stomach. I therefore applied myself diligently to discover what kinds of food suited me best. But, first, I resolved to try, whether those, which pleased my palate, agreed or disagreed with my stomach, in order to judge for myself of the truth of that proverb, which I once held true, and is universally held as such in the highest degree, insomuch that epicures, who give a loose to their appetites, lay it down as a fundamental maxim. This proverb is, that whatever pleases the palate, must agree with the stomach, and nourish the body; or whatever is palatable must be equally wholesome and nourishing. The issue was, that I found it to be false: for, though rough and very cold wines, as likewise melons and other fruits, sallad, fish and pork, tarts, garden-stuff, pastry, and the like, were very pleasing to my palate, the disagreed with me notwithstanding. Having convinced myself, that the proverb in question was false, I look'd upon it as such; and, taught by experience, I gave over the use of such meats and wines, and likewise of ice; chose wine suited to my stomach, drinking of it but the quantity I knew I could digest. I did the same by my meat, as well in regard to quantity as to quality, accustoming myself never to cloy my stomach with eating or drinking; but constantly rise from table with a disposition to eat and drink still more. In this I conformed to the proverb, which says, that a man, to consult his health, must check his appetite. Having in this manner, and for these reasons, conquered intemperance and irregularity, I betook myself intirely to a temperate and regular life: which effected in me the alteration already mentioned, that is, in less than a year it rid me of all those disorders, which had taken so deep a root in me; nay, as I have already observed, had made such a progress, as to be in a manner incurable. It had likewise this other good effect, that I no longer experienced those annual fits of sickness, with which I used to be afflicted, while I followed a different, that is a sensual, course of life; for then I used to be attacked every year with a strange kind of fever, which sometimes brought me to death's door. From this disease, then, I also freed myself, and became exceeding healthy, as I have continued from that time forward to this very day; and for no other reason than that I never trespassed against regularity, which by its infinite efficacy has been the cause, that the meat I constantly eat, and the wine I constantly drink, being such as agreed with my constitution, and taken in proper quantities, imparted all their virtue to my body, and then left it without difficulty, and without engendering in it any bad humours.

In consequence therfore of my taking such methods, I have always enjoyed, and (God be praised) actually enjoy, the best of healths. It is true, indeed, that, besides the two forgoing most important rules relative to eating and drinking, which I have ever been very scrupulous to observe; that is, not to take of any thing, but as much as my stomach can easily digest, and to use those things only, which agree with me; I have carefully avoided heat, cold, and extraordinary fatigue, interruption of my usual hours of rest, excessive venery, making any stay in bad air, and exposing myself to the wind and sun; for these, too, are great disorders. But then, fortunately, there is no great difficulty in avoiding them, the love of life and health having more sway over men of understanding, than any satisfaction they could find in doing what must be extremely hurtful to their constitution. I have likewise done all that lay in my power to avoid those evils, which we do not find so easy to remove; these are melancholy, hatred, and other violent passions, which appear to have the greatest influence over our bodies. However, I have not been able to guard so well against either one or the other kind of these disorders, as not to suffer myself now and then to be hurried away by many, not to say, all of them; but I have reaped the benefit of knowing by experience that these passions have, in the main, no great influence over bodies governed by the two foregoing rules of eating and drinking, and therefore can do them but very little harm; so that it may with great truth be affirmed, that whoever observes these two capital rules, is liable to very little inconveniency from any other excesses. This, Galen, who was an eminent physician, observed before me. He affirms, that so long as he followed these rules relative to eating and drinking, he suffered but little from other disorders, so little, that they never gave him above a day's uneasiness. That what he says is true, I am a living witness, and so are many others, who know me, and have seen, how often I have been exposed to heats and colds, and such other disagreeable changes of weather; and have, likewise, seen me (owing to various misfortunes, which have more than once befallen me) greatly disturbed my mind. For they can not only say of me, that such disturbance of mind has done me very little harm, but they can aver of many others, who did not lead a sober and regular life, that it proved very prejudicial to them, amongst whom was a brother of my own, and others of my family, who trusting to the goodness of their constitution, did not follow my way of living. The consequence hereof was a great misfortune to them, the perturbations of the mind having thereby acquired an extraordinary influence over their bodies. Such, in a word, was their grief and dejection at seeing me involved in expensive law-suits, commenced against my by great and powerful men, that, fearing I should be cast, they were seized with that melancholy humour, with which intemperate bodies always abound; and these humours had such an influence over them, and increased to such a degree, as to carry them off before their time; whereas I suffered nothing on the occasion, as I had in me no superfluous humours of that kind. Nay, in order to keep up my spirits, I brought myself to think, that God had raised up these suits against me, in order to make me more sensible of my strength of body and mind; and that I should get the better of them with honour and advantage, as it, in fact, came to pass: for, at last, I obtained a decree exceeding favourable to my fortune and my character, which, though it gave me the highest pleasure, had not the power to do me any harm in other respects. Thus it is plain, that neither melancholy nor any other affection of the mind can hurt bodies governed with temperance and regularity.

But I must go a step further, and say, that even misfortunes themselves can do but very little mischief, or cause but very little pain, to such bodies; and that this is true, I have myself experienced at the age of seventy. I happened, as is often the case, to be in a coach, which going at a pretty smart rate, was overset, and in that condition drawn a considerable way by the horses, before means could be found to stop them; whence I received so many shocks and bruises, that I was taken out with my head and all the rest of my body terribly battered, and a dislocated leg and arm. When I was brought home, the family immediately sent for the physicians, who, on their arrival, seeing me in so bad a plight, concluded, that within three days I should die; nevertheless, they would try what good two things would do me; one was to bleed me, the other to purge me; and thereby prevent my humours altering, as they every moment expected, to such a degree, as to ferment greatly, and bring on a high fever. But I, on the contrary, who knew, that the sober life I had led for many years past, had so well united, harmonized, and disposed my humours, as not to leave it in their power to ferment to such a degree, refused to be either bled, or purged. I just caused my leg and arm to be set, an suffered myself to be rubbed with some oils, which they said were proper on the occasion. Thus, without using any other kind of remedy, I recovered, as I thought I should, without feeling the least alteration in myself, or any other bad effects from the accident; a thing, which appeared miraculous even in the eyes of the physicians. Hence we are to infer, that whoever leads a sober and regular life, and commits no excess in his diet, can suffer but very little from disorders of any other kind, or external accidents. On the contrary, I conclude, especially from the late trial I have had, that excesses in eating and drinking are fatal. Of this I convinced myself four years ago, when by the advice of my physicians, the instigation of my friends, and the importunity of my own family, I consented to such an excess, which, as it will appear hereafter, was attended with far worse consequences, than could naturally be expected. This excess consisted in increasing the quantity of food I generally made use of; which increase alone brought me to a most cruel fit of sickness. And as it is a case so much in point to the subject in hand, and the knowledge of it may be useful to some of my readers, I shall take the trouble to relate it.

I say, then, that my dearest friends and relations, actuated by the warm and laudable affection and regard they have for me, seeing how little I eat, represented to me, in conjunction with my physicians, that the sustenance I took could not be sufficient to support one so far advanced in years, when it was become necessary not only to preserve nature, but to increase its vigour. That, as this could not be done without food, it was absolutely incumbent upon me to eat a little more plentifully. I, on the other hand, produced my reasons for not complying with their desires. These were, that nature is content with little, and that with this little I had preserved myself so many years; and that, to me, the habit of it was become a second nature; and that it was more agreeable to reason, that, as I advanced in years and lost my strength, I should rather lessen than increase the quantity of my food: Farther, that it was but natural to think, that the powers of the stomach grew weaker from day to day; on which account I could see no reason to make such an addition. To corroborate my arguments, I alleged that those two natural and very true proverbs; one, that he, who has a mind to eat a great deal, must eat but little; which is said for no other reason than this, that eating little makes a man live very long, and living very long he must eat a great deal. The other proverb was, that what we leave after making a hearty meal, does us more good than what we have eat. But neither these proverbs, nor any other arguments I could think of, were able to prevent their teazing me more than ever. Wherefore, not to appear obstinate, or affect to know more than the physicians themselves; but, above all, to please my family, who very earnestly desired it, from a persuasion that such an addition to my usual allowance would preserve my strength, I consented to increase the quantity of food, but with two ounces only. So that, as before, what with bread, meat, the yolk of an egg, and soup, I eat as much, as weighed in all twelve ounces, neither more nor less, I now increased it to fourteen; and as before I drank but fourteen ounces of wine, I now increased it to sixteen. This increase and irregularity, had, in eight days time, such an effect upon me, that, from being chearful and brisk, I began to be peevish and melancholy, so that nothing could please me; and was constantly so strangely disposed, that I neither knew what to say to others, nor what to do with myself. On the twelfth day, I was attacked with a most violent pain in my side, which held me twenty-two hours, and was succeeded by a terrible fever, which continued thirty-five days and as many nights, without giving me a moment's respite; though, to say the truth, it began to abate gradually on the fifteenth. But notwithstanding such abatement, I could not, during the whole time, sleep half a quarter of an hour together, insomuch that every one looked upon me as a dead man. But, God be praised, I recovered merely by my former regular course of life, though then in my seventy-eighth year, and in the coldest season of a very cold year, and reduced to a mere skeleton; and I am positive that it was the great regularity I had observed for so many years, and that only, which rescued me from the jaws of death. In all that time I never knew what sickness was, unless I may call by that same name some slight indispositions of a day or two's continuance; the regular life I had led, as I have already taken notice, for so many years, not having permitted any superfluous or bad humours to breed in me; or if they did, to acquire such strength and malignity, a they generally acquire in the superannuated bodies of those, who live without rule. And as there was not any old malignity in my humours (which is the thing that kills people) but only that, which my new irregularity had occasioned, this fit of sickness, though exceeding violent, had not the strength to destroy me. This it was, and nothing else, that saved my life; whence may be gathered, how great is the power and efficacy of regularity; and how great, likewise, is that of irregularity, which in a few days could bring on me so terrible a fit of sickness, just as regularity had preserved me in health for so many years.

And it appears to me a no weak argument, that, since the world, consisting of the four elements, is upheld by order; and our life, as to the body, is no other than a harmonious combination of the same four elements, so it should be preserved and maintained by the very same order; and, on the other hand, it must be worn out by sickness, or destroyed by death, which are produced by the contrary effects. By order the arts are more easily learned; by order armies are rendered victorious; by order, in a word, families, cities, and even states are maintained. Hence I concluded, that orderly living is no other than a most certain cause and foundation of health and long life; nay I cannot help saying, that it is the only and true medicine; and whoever weighs the matter well, must also conclude, that this is really the case. Hence it is, that when a physician comes to visit a patient, the first thing he prescribes, is to live regularly. In like manner, when a physician takes leave of a patient, on his being recovered, he advises him, as he tenders his health, to lead a regular life. And it is not to be doubted, that, were a patient so recovered to live in that manner, he could never be sick again, as it removes every cause of illness; and so, for the future, would never want either physician or physic. Nay, by attending duly to what I have said, he would become his own physician, and, indeed, the best he could have; since, in fact, no many can be a perfect physician to any one but himself. The reason of which is, that any man may, by repeated trials, acquire a perfect knowledge of his own constitution, and the most hidden qualities of his body; and what wine and food agree with his stomach. Now, it is so far from being an easy matter to know these things perfectly of another, that we cannot without much trouble discover them in ourselves, since a great deal of time and repeated trials are requisite for the purpose.

These trials are, indeed, (if I may say it) more than necessary, as there is a greater variety in the natures and constitutions of different men, than in their persons. Who could believe, that old wine, wine that had passed its first year, should disagree with my stomach, and new wine agree with it? and that pepper, which is looked upon as a warm spice, should not have a warm effect upon me, insomuch that I find myself more warmed and comforted by cinnamon? Where is the physician, that could have informed me of these two latent qualities, since I myself, even by a long course of observation, could scarce discover them? From all these reasons it follows, that it is impossible to be a perfect physician to another. Since, therefore, a man cannot have a better physician than himself, nor any physic better than a regular life, a regular life he ought to embrace.

I do not, however, mean, that, for the knowledge and cure of such disorders, as often befall those who do not live regularly, there is no occasion for a physician, and that his assistance ought to be slighted. For, if we are apt to receive such great comfort from friends, who come to visit us in our illness, though they do no more than testify their concern for us, and bid us be of good cheer; how much more regard ought we to have for the physician, who is a friend that comes to see us in order to relieve us, and promises us a cure? But for the bare purpose of keeping ourselves in good health, I am of the opinion, that we should consider as a physician this regular life, which, as we have seen, is our natural and proper physic, since it preserves men, even those of a bad constitution, in health; makes them live sound and hearty to the age of one hundred and upwards; and prevents their dying of sickness, or through a corruption of their humours, but merely by a dissolution of their radical moisture, when quite exhausted; all which effects several wise men have attributed to potable gold, and the elixir, sought for by many, but discovered by few. However to confess the truth, men, for the most part, are very sensual and intemperate, and love to satisfy their appetites, and to commit every excess; therefore, seeing that they cannot avoid being greatly injured by such excess, as often as they are guilty of it, they, by way of apologizing for their conduct, say, that it is better to live ten years less, and enjoy themselves; not considering, of what importance are ten years more of life, especially a healthy life, and at a maturer age; when men become sensible of their progress in knowledge and virtue, which cannot attain to any degree of perfection before this period of life.

Not to speak, at present, of many other advantages, I shall barely mention that in regard to letters and the sciences; far the greatest number of the best and most celebrated books extant, were written during that period of life, and those ten years, which some make it their business to undervalue, in order to give a loose to their appetites. Be that as it will, I would not act like them. I rather coveted to live these ten years, and, had I not done so, I should never have finished those tracts, which I have composed in consequence of my having been sound and hearty these ten years past; and which I have the pleasure to think will be of service to others. These sensualists add, that a regular life is such as no man can lead. To this I answer, Galen, who was so great a physician, led such a life, and chose it as the best physic. The same did Plato, Cicero, Isocrates, and many other great men of former times; whom, not to tire the reader, I shall forbear naming: and, in our own days, pope Paul Farnese led it, and cardinal Bembo; and it was for that reason they lived so long; likewise our two doges, Lando and Donato; besides many others of meaner condition, and those who live not only in cities, but also in different parts of the country, who all found great benefit by conforming to this regularity. Therefore, since many have led this life, and many actually lead it, it is not such a life but that every one may conform to it; and the more so, as no great difficulty attends it; nothing, indeed, being requisite but to begin in good earnest, as the above-mentioned Cicero affirms, and all those who now live in this manner. Plato, you will say, though he himself lived very regularly, affirms, notwithstanding, that, in republics, men cannot do so, being often obliged to expose themselves to heat, cold, and several other kinds of hardship, and other things, which are all so many disorders, and incompatable with a regular life. I answer, as I have already observed, that these are not disorders attended with any bad consequence, or which affect either health or life, when the man, who undergoes them, observes the rules of sobriety, and commits no excess in the two points concerning diet, which a republican may very well avoid, nay it is requisite he should avoid; because, by so doing, he may be sure either to escape those disorders, which, otherwise, it would be no easy matter for him to escape while exposed to these hardships; or, in case he could not escape them, he may more easily and speedily prevent their bad effects.

Here it may be objected, and some actually object, that he, who leads a regular life, having constantly, when well, made use of food fit for the sick, and in small quantities, has no resource left in case of illness. To this I might, in the first place, answer, that nature, desirous to preserve man in good health as long as possible, informs him, herself, how he is to act in time of illness; for she immediately deprives him, when sick, of his appetite, in order that he may eat but little; because nature (as I have said already) is satisfied with little; wherefore, it is requisite, that a man, when sick, whether he has been a regular or irregular liver, should use no meats, but such as are suited to his disorder; and of these even in a much smaller quantity than he was wont to do, when in health. For were he to eat as much as he used to do, he would die by it; because it would be only adding to the burden, with which nature was already oppressed, by giving her a greater quantity of food, than she can in such circumstances support; and this, I imagine, would be a sufficient caution to any sick person. But, independent of all this, I might answer some others, and still better, that whoever leads a regular life, cannot be sick; or, at least, but seldom, and for a short time; because, by living regularly, he extirpates every seed of sickness; and thus, by removing the cause, prevents the effect; so that he, who pursues a regular course of life, need not be apprehensive of illness, as he need not be afraid of the effect, who has guarded against the cause.

Since it therefore appears that a regular life is so profitable and virtuous, so lovely and so holy, it ought to be universally followed and embraced; and more so, as it does not clash with the means or duties of any station, but is easy to all; because, to lead it, a man need not tie himself down to eat so little as I do, or not to eat fruit, fish, and other things of that kind, from which I abstain, who eat little, because it is sufficient for my puny and weak stomach; and fruit, fish, and other things of that kind, disagree with me, which is my reason for not touching them. Those, however, with whom such things agree, may, and ought to eat of them; since they are not by any means forbid the use use of such sustinance. But, then, both they, and all others, are forbid to eat a greater quantity of any kind of food, even of that which agrees with them, than what their stomachs can easily digest; the same is to be understood of drink. Hence it is that those, with whom nothing disagrees, are not bound to observe any rule but that relating to the quantity, and not to the quality, of their food; a rule which they may, without the least difficulty in the world, comply with.

Let nobody tell me, that there are numbers, who, though they live most irregularly, live in health and spirits, to those remote periods of life, attained by the most sober; for, this argument being grounded on a case full of uncertainty and hazard, and which, besides, so seldom occurs, as to look more like a miracle than the work of nature, men should not suffer themselves to be thereby persuaded to live irregularly, nature having been too liberal to those, who did so without suffering by it; a favour, which very few have any right to expect. Whoever, trusting to his youth, or the strength of his constitution, or the goodness of his stomach, slights these observations, must expect to suffer greatly by so doing, and live in constant danger of disease and death. I therefore affirm, that an old man, even of a bad constitution, who leads a regular and sober life, is surer of a long one, than a young man of the best constitution, who leads a disorderly life. It is not to be doubted, however, that a man blessed with a good constitution may, by living temperately, expect to live longer than one, whose constitution is not so good; and that God and nature can dispose matters so, that a man shall bring into the world with him so sound a constitution, as to live long and healthy, without observing such strick rules; and then die in a very advanced age through a mere dissolution of his elementary parts; as was the case, in Venice, of the procurator Thomas Contarini; and in Padua, of the cavalier Antonio Capo di Vacca. But it is not one man in a hundred thousand, that so much can be said of. If others have a mind to live long and healthy, and die without sickness of body or mind, but by mere dissolution, they must submit to live regularly, since the cannot otherwise expect to enjoy the fruits of such a life, which are almost infinite in number, and each of them, in particular, of infinite value. For, as such regularity keeps the humours of the body cleansed and purified; it suffers no vapors to ascend from the stomach to the head; hence the brain of him, who lives in that manner, enjoys such a constant serenity, that he is always perfectly master of himself. He, therefore, easily soars above the low and groveling concerns of this life, to the exalted and beautiful contemplation of heavenly things, to his exceeding great comfort and satisfaction; because he, by this means, comes to consider, know, and understand that, which otherwise he would never have considered, known, or understood; that is, how great is the power, wisdom, and goodness of the Deity. He then descends into nature, and acknowledges her for the daughter of God; and sees, and even feels with his hands, that, which in any other age, or with a perception less clear, he could never have seen or felt. He then truly discerns the brutality of that vice into which they fall, who know not how to subdue their passions, and those three importunate lusts, which, one would imagine, came all together into the world with us, in order to keep us in perpetual anxiety and disturbance. These are, the lust of the flesh, the lust of honours, and the lust of riches; which are apt to increase with years in such old persons as do not lead a regular life; because, in their passage through the stage of manhood, they did not, as they ought, renounce sensuality and their passions; and take up with sobriety and reason; virtues which men of a regular life, did not neglect when they passed through the above-mentioned stage. For, knowing such passions are such lusts to be inconsistent with reason, by which they are entirely governed; they, at once, broke loose from all temptations to vice; and, instead of being slaves to their inordinate appetites, they applied themselves to virtue and good works; and by these means, they altered their conduct, and became men of good and sober lives. When, therefore, in process of time, they see themselves brought by a long series of years to their dissolution, conscious that, through the singular mercy of God, they had so sincerely relinquished the paths of vice, as never afterwards to enter them; and moreover hoping, through the merits of our Saviour Jesus Christ, to die in his favour, they do not suffer themselves to be cast down at the thoughts of death, knowing that they must die. This is particularly the case, when, loaded with honour, and sated with life, they see themselves arrived at that age, which not one in many thousands of those, who live otherwise, ever attains. They have still the greater reason not to be dejected at the thoughts of death, as it does not attack them violently and by surprize, with a bitter and painful turn of their humours, with feverish sensations, and sharp pains, but steals upon them insensibly and with the greatest ease and gentleness; such an end, proceeding intirely from an exhaustion of the radical moisture, which decays by degrees like the oil of a lamp; so that they pass gently, without any sickness, from this terrestrial and mortal to a celestial and eternal life.

O holy and truly happy regularity! How holy and happy should men, in fact, deem thee, since the opposite habit is the cause of such guilt and misery, as evidently appears to those who consider the opposite effects of both! so that men should know thee by thy voice alone, and thy lovely name; for what a glorious name, what a noble thing, is an orderly and sober life! as, on the contrary, the bare mention of disorder and intemperance is offensive to our ears. Nay, there is the same difference between the mentioning these two things, as between the uttering of the words angel and devil.

Thus I have assigned my reasons for abandoning intemperance, and betaking myself intirely to a sober life; with the method I pursued in doing so, and what was the consequence of it; and, finally, the advantages an blessings, which a sober life confers upon those who embrace it. Some sensual, inconsiderate persons affirm, that a long life is no blessing; and that the state of a man, who has passed his seventy-fifth year, cannot really be called life, but death: but this is a great mistake, as I shall fully prove; and it is my sincere wish, that all men would endeavour to attain my old age, in order that they too may enjoy that period of life, which of all others is the most desirable.

I will therefore give an account of my recreations, and the relish which I find at this stage of life, in order to convince the public (which may likewise be done by all those who know me) that the state I have now attained to is by no means death, but real life; such a life, as by many is deemed happy, since it abounds with all the felicity that can be enjoyed in this world. And this testimony they will give, in the first place, because they see, and not without the greatest amazement, the good state of health and spirits I enjoy; how I mount my horse without any assistance, or advantage of situation; and how I not only ascend a single flight of stairs, but climb up an hill from bottom to top, afoot, and with the greatest of ease and unconcern; then how gay, pleasant, and good-humoured I am; how free from every perturbation of mind, and every disagreeable thought; in lieu of which, joy and peace have so firmly fixed their residence in my bosom, as never to depart from it. Moreover, they know in what manner I pass my time, so as not to find life a burden; seeing I can contrive to spend every hour of it with the greatest delight and pleasure, having frequent opportunities of conversing with many honourable gentlemen, men valuable for their good sense and manners, their acquaintance with letters, and every other good quality. Then, when I cannot enjoy their conversation, I betake myself to the reading of some good book. When I have read as much as I like, I write; endeavouring, in this as in everything else, to be of service to others, to the utmost of my power. And all these things I do with the greatest ease to myself, at their proper seasons, and in my own house; which, besides being situated in the most beautiful quarter of this noble and learned city of Padua, is, in itself, really convenient and handsome, such, in a word, as it is no longer the fashion to build; for, in one part of it, I can shelter myself from extreme heat; and, in the other, from extreme cold, having contrived the apartments according to the rules of architecture, which teach us what is to be observed in practice. Besides this house, I have my several gardens, supplied with running waters; and in which I always find something to do, that amuses me. I have another way of diverting myself, which is going every April and May; and, likewise, every September and October, for some days, to enjoy an eminence belonging to me in the Euganean mountains, and in the most beautiful part of them, adorned with fountains and gardens; and, above all, a convenient and handsome lodge; in which place I likewise now and then make one in some hunting party suitable to my taste and age. Then I enjoy for as many days my villa in the plain, which is laid out in regular streets, all terminating in a large square, in the middle of which stands a church, suited to the condition of the place. This villa is divided by a wide and rapid branch of the river Brenta, on both sides of which there is a considerable extent of country, consisting intirely of fertile and well-cultivated fields. Besides, this district is now, God be praised, exceedingly well inhabited, which it was not at first, but rather the reverse; for it was marshy; and the air so unwholesome, as to make it a residence fitter for snakes than men. But, on my draining off the waters, the air mended, and people resorted to it so fast, and increased to such a degree, that it soon acquired the perfection in which it now appears: hence, I may say with truth, that I have offered this place, an alter and a temple to God, with souls to adore him: these are things which afford me infinite pleasure, comfort, and satisfaction, as often as I go to see and enjoy them.

At the same seasons every year, I revisit some of the neighbouring cities, and enjoy such of my friends as live there, taking the greatest pleasure in their company and conversation; and by their means I also enjoy the conversation of other men of parts, who live in the same places; such as architects, painters, sculptors, musicians, and husbandmen, with whom this age certainly abounds. I visit their new works; I revisit their former ones; and I always learn something, which gives me satisfaction. I see palaces, gardens, antiquities; and with these, the squares and other public places, the churches, the fortifications, leaving nothing unobserved, from whence I may reap either entertainment or instruction. But what delights me most, is, in my journies backwards and forwards, to contemplate the situation and other beauties of the places I pass through; some in the plain, others on hills, adjoining to rivers or fountains; with a great many fine houses and gardens. Nor are my recreations rendered less agreeable and entertaining by my not feeling well, or not hearing readily every thing that is said to me; or by any other of my faculties not being perfect; for they are all, thank God, in the highest perfection; particularly my palate, which now relishes better the simple fare I eat, wherever I happen to be, than it formerly did with the most delicate dishes, when I led an irregular life. Nor does the change of beds give me any uneasiness, so that I sleep every where soundly and quietly, without experiencing the least disturbance; and all my dreams are pleasant and delightful.

It is likewise with the greatest pleasure and satisfaction I behold the success of an undertaking so important to this state, I mean that of draining and improving so many uncultivated pieces of ground, an undertaking begun within my memory; and which I never thought I should live to see compleated; knowing how slow republics are apt to proceed in enterprises of great importance. Nevertheless, I have lived to see it; and was even in person, in the marshy places, along with those appointed to superintend the draining of them, for two months together, during the greatest heats of summer, without ever finding myself the worse for the fatigues of inconveniences I suffered; of so much efficacy is that orderly life, which I every where constantly lead.

What is more, I am in the greatest hopes, or rather sure, to see the beginning and completion of another undertaking of no less importance, which is that of preserving our estuary or port, that last and wonderful bulwark of my dear country, the preservation of which (it is not to flatter my vanity to say it, but merely to do justice to the truth) has been more than once recommended by me to this republic, by word of mouth, and in writings which cost me many nights study. And to this dear country of mine, as I am bound by the laws of nature to do every thing, from which it may reap any benefit, so I most ardently wish perpetual duration, and a long succession of every kind of prosperity. Such are my genuine and no trifling satisfactions; such are the recreations and diversions of my old age, which is so much the more to be valued than the old age, or even youth, of other men, because being freed, by God's grace, from the perturbations of the mind, and the infirmities of the body, it no longer experiences any of those contrary emotions, which torment a number of young men, and many old ones destitute of strength and health, and every other blessing.

And if it be lawful to compare little matters, and such as are esteemed trifling, to affairs of importance, I will further venture to say, that such are the effects of this sober life, that at my present age of eighty-three, I have been able to write a very entertaining comedy, abounding with innocent mirth and pleasant jests. This species of composition is generally the child and offspring of youth, as tragedy is that of old age; the former being by its facetious and sprightly turn suited to the bloom of life, and the latter by its gravity adapted to riper years. Now, if that good old man [Sophocles], a Grecian by birth, and a poet, was so much extolled for having written a tragedy at the age of seventy-three, and, on that account alone, reputed of sound memory and understanding, though tragedy be a grave and melancholy poem; why should I be deemed less happy, and to have a smaller share of memory and understanding, who have, at an age, ten years more advanced than his, written a comedy, which, as every one knows, is a merry and pleasant kind of composition? And, indeed, if I may be allowed to be an impartial judge in my own cause, I cannot help thinking, that I am now of sounder memory and understanding, and heartier, than hew was when ten years younger.

And, that no comfort might be wanting to the fulness of my years, whereby my great age may be rendered less irksome, or rather the number of my enjoyments increased, I have the additional comfort of seeing a kind of immortality in a succession of descendants. For, as often as I return home, I find there, before me, not one or two, but eleven grandchildren, the oldest of them eighteen, and the youngest two; all the offspring of one father and one mother; all blessed with the best health; and, by what as yet appears, fond of learning, and of good parts and morals. Some of the youngest I always play with; and, indeed, children from three to five are only fit for play. Those above that age I make companions of; and, as nature has bestowed very fine voices upon them, I amuse myself, besides, with seeing and hearing them sing, and play on various instruments. Nay, I sing myself, as I have a better voice now, and a clearer and louder pipe, than at any other period of life. Such are the recreations of my old age.

Whence it appears, that the life I lead is chearful, and not gloomy, as some persons pretend, who know no better; to whom, in order that it may appear what value I set on every other kind of life, I must declare, that I would not exchange my manner of living or my grey hairs with any of those young men, even of the best constitution, who give way to their appetites; knowing, as I do, that such are daily, nay hourly, subject, as I have observed, to a thousand kind of ailments and deaths. This is, in fact, so obvious, as to require no proof. Nay, I remember perfectly well, how I used to behave at that time of life. I know how inconsiderately that age is apt to act, and how foolhardy young men, hurried on by the heat of their blood, are wont to be; how apt they are to presume too much on their own strength in all their actions; and how sanguine they are in their expectations; as well on account of the little experience they have had for the the time past, as by reason of the power they enjoy in their own imaginations over the time to come. Hence they expose themselves rashly to every kind of danger; and, banishing reason, and bowing their necks to the yoke of concupiscence, endeavour to gratify all their appetites, not minding, fools as they are, that they thereby hasten, as I have several times observed, the approach of what they would most willingly avoid, I mean sickness, and death. Of these two evils, one is troublesome and painful, the other, above all things, dreadful and insupportable; insupportable to every man, who has given himself up to his sensual appetites, and to young men in particular, to whom it appears a hardship to die an early death; dreadful to those, who reflect on the errors, to which this mortal life is subject, and on the vengeance, which the justice of God is wont to take on sinners, by condemning them to everlasting punishment. On the other hand, I, in my old age (praise to the Almighty) am exempt from both these apprehensions; from the one, because I am sure and certain, that I cannot fall sick, having removed all the causes of illness by my divine medicine; from the other, that of death, because from so many years experience I have learned to obey reason; whence I not only think it a great piece of folly to fear that, which cannot be avoided, but likewise firmly expect some consolation, from the grace of Jesus Christ, when I shall arrive at that period.

Besides, though I am sensible that I must, like others, reach that term, it is yet at so great a distance, that I cannot discern it, because I know I shall not die except by mere dissolution, having already, by my regular course of life, shut up all the other avenues of death, and thereby prevented the humours of my body from making any other war upon me, than that which I must expect from the elements employed in the composition of this mortal frame. I am not so simple as not to know, that, as I was born, so I must die. But that is a desirable death, which nature brings on us by way of dissolution. For nature, having herself formed the union between our body and soul, knows best in what manner it may be most easily dissolved, and grants us a longer day to do it, than we could expect from sickness, which is violent. This is the death, which, without speaking like a poet, I may call, not death, but life. Nor can it be otherwise. Such a death does not overtake one till after a very long course of years, and in consequence of an extreme weakness; it being only by slow degrees, that men grow too feeble to walk, and unable to reason, becoming blind, and deaf, decrepid, and full of every other kind of infirmity. Now I (by God's blessing) may be quite sure that I am at a very great distance from such a period. Nay, I have reason to think, that my soul, having so agreeable a dwelling in my body, as not to meet with any thing in it but peace, love, and harmony, not only between its humours, but between my reason and my senses, is exceedingly content and well pleased with her present situation: and of course, that a great length of time and many years must be requisite to dislodge her. Whence it must be concluded for certain, that I have still a series of years to live in health and spirits, and enjoy this beautiful world, which is, indeed, beautiful to those, who know how to make it so, as I have done, and likewise expect to be able to do, with God's assistance, in the next; and all by the means of virtue, and that divine regularity of life, which I have adopted, concluding an alliance with my reason, and declaring war against my sensual appetites; a thing which every man may do, who desired to live as he ought.

Now, if this sober life be so happy; if its name be so desirable and delightful; if the possession of the blessings which attend it, be so stable and permanent, all I have still left to do, is to beseech (since I cannot compass my desires by the powers of oratory) every man of a liberal disposition, and sound understanding, to embrace with open arms this most valuable treasure of a long and healthy life; a treasure, which as it exceeds all the other riches and blessings of this world, so it deserves above all things to be cherished, sought after, and carefully preserved. This is that divine sobriety, agreeable to the Deity, the friend of nature, the daughter of reason, the sister of all the virtues, the companion of temperate living, modest, courteous, content with little, regular, and perfect mistress of all her operations. From her, as from their proper root, spring life, health, chearfulness, industry, learning, and all those actions and employments worth of noble and generous minds. The laws of God and man are all in her favour. Repletion, excess, intemperance, superfluous humours, diseases, fevers, pains, and the dangers of death, vanish, in her presence, like clouds before the sun. Her comeliness ravishes every well-disposed mind. Her influence is so sure, as to promise to all a very long and agreeable existence; the facility of acquiring her is such, as ought to induce every one to look for her, and share in her victories. And, lastly, she promises to be a mild and agreeable guardian of life; as well of the rich as of the poor; of the male as of the female sex; the old as of the young; being that, which teaches the rich modesty; the poor frugality; men, continence; women, chastity; the old, how to ward off the attacks of death; and bestows on youth firmer and securer hopes of life. Sobriety renders the senses clear, the body light, the understanding lively, the soul brisk, the memory tenacious, our motions free, and all our actions regular and easy. By means of sobriety, the soul delivered, as it were, of her earthly burthen, experiences a great deal of her natural liberty: the spirits circulate gently through the arteries; the blood runs freely through the veins; the heat of the body, kept mild and temperate, has mild and temperate effects: and, lastly, our faculties, being under a perfect regulation, preserves a pleasing and agreeable harmony.

O most innocent and holy sobriety, the sole refreshment of nature, the nursing mother of human life, the true physic of soul as well as of body. How ought men to praise thee, and thank thee for thy princely gifts! since thou bestowest on them the means of preserving this blessing, I mean life and health, than which it has not pleased God we should enjoy a greater on this side of the grave, life and existence being a thing so naturally coveted, and willingly preserved, by every living creature. But, as I do not intend to write a panegyric on this rare and excellent virtue, I shall put an end to this discourse, lest I should be guilty of excess, in dwelling so long on so pleasing a subject. Yet as numberless things may still be said of it, I leave off, with an intention of setting forth the rest of its praises at a more convenient opportunity.

A COMPENDIUM OF A SOBER LIFE

My treatise on a sober life has begun to answer my desire, in being of service to many persons born with a weak constitution, who every time they committed the least excess, found themselves greatly indisposed, a thing which it must be allowed does not happen to robust people: several of these persons of weak constitutions, on seeing the foregoing treatise, have betaken themselves to a regular course of life, convinced by experience of its utility. In like manner, I should be glad to be of service to those, who are born with a good constitution, and presuming upon it, lead a disorderly life; whence it comes to pass, that, on their attaining the age of sixty or thereabouts, they are attacked with various pains and diseases; some with the gout, some with pains in the side, and others with pains in the stomach, and the like, to which they would not be subject, were they to embrace a sober life; and as most of them die before they attain their eightieth year, they would live to a hundred, the time allowed to man by God and nature. And, it is but reasonable to believe, that the intention of this our mother is, that we should all attain that term, in order that we might all taste the sweets of every state of life. But, as our birth is subject to the revolution of the heavens, these have great influence over it, especially in rendering our constitutions robust or infirm; a thing, which nature cannot ward against; for, if she could, we should all bring a good constitution with us into the world. But then she hopes, that man, being endowed with reason and understanding, may of himself compensate, by dint of art, the want of that, which the heavens have denied him; and, by means of a sober life, contrive to mend his infirm constitution, live to a great age, and always enjoy good health.

For man, it is not to be doubted, may by art exempt himself in part from the influence of the heavens; it being common opinion, that the heavens give an inclination, but do not impel us; for which reason the learned say, that a wise man rules the stars. I was born with a very choleric disposition, insomuch that there was no living with me; but I took notice of it, and considered, that a person swayed by his passion, must at certain times be no better than a madman; I mean at those times, when he suffers his passions to predominate, because he then renounces his reason and understanding. I, therefore, resolved to make my choleric disposition give way to reason; so that now, though born choleric, I never suffer anger intirely to overcome me. The man, who is naturally of a bad constitution, may, in like manner, by dint of reason, and a sober life, live to a great age and in good health, as I have done, who had naturally the worst, so that it was impossible I should live above forty years, whereas I now find myself sound and hearty at the age of eighty-six; and were it not for the long and violent fits of illness which I experienced in my youth to such a degree, that the physicians gave me over, and which robbed me of my radical moisture, a loss absolutely irreparable, I might expect to attain the abovementioned term of one hundred. But I know for good reasons that it is impossible; and, therefore, do not think of it. It is enough for me, that I have lived forty-six years beyond the term I had a right to expect; and that, during this so long a respite, all my senses have continued perfect; and even my teeth, my voice, my memory, and my strength. But what is still more, my brain is more itself now than it ever was; nor do any of these powers abate as I advance in years; and this because, as I grow older, I lessen the quantity of my solid food.

This retrenchment is necessary, nor can it be avoided, since it is impossible for a man to live for ever; and, as he draws near his end, he is reduced so low as to be no longer able to take any nourishment, unless it be to swallow, and that too with difficulty, the yolk of an egg in the four and twenty hours, and thus end by mere dissolution, without any pain or sickness, as I expect will be my case. This is a blessing of great importance; yet may be expected by all those, who shall lead a sober life, of whatever degree or condition, whether high, or middling, or low; for we are all of the same species, and composed of the same four elements. And, since a long and healthy life ought to be greatly coveted by every man, as I shall presently shew, I conclude, that every man is bound in duty to exert himself to obtain longevity, and that he cannot promise himself such a blessing without temperance and sobriety.

Some allege, that many, without leading such a life, have lived to an hundred, and that in constant health, though they eat a great deal, and used indiscriminately every kinds of viands and wine; and, therefore, flatter themselves, that they shall be equally fortunate. But in this they are guilty of two mistakes; the first is, that it is not one in an hundred thousand that ever attains that happiness; the other mistake is, that such, in the end, most assuredly contract some illness, which carries them off: nor can they ever be sure of ending their days otherwise: so that the safest way to obtain a long and healthy life is, at least after forty, to embrace sobriety. This is no such difficult affair, since history informs us of so many who in former times lived with the greatest temperance; and I know that the present age furnishes us with many such instances, reckoning myself one of the number: we are all human beings, and endowed with reason, consequently we are masters of our actions.

This sobriety is reduced to two things, quality and quantity. The first, namely quality, consists in nothing, but not eating food, or drinking wines, prejudicial to the stomach. The second, which is quantity, consists in not eating or drinking more than the stomach can easily digest; which quantity and quality every man should be a perfect judge of by the time he is forty, or fifty, or sixty; and, whoever observes these two rules, may be said to live a regular and sober life. This is of so much virtue and efficacy, that the humours of such a man's body become most homogeneous, harmonious, and perfect; and, when thus improved, are no longer liable to be corrupted or disturbed by any other disorders whatsoever, such as suffering excessive heat or cold, too much fatigue, want of natural rest, and the like, unless in the last degree of excess. Wherefore, since the humours of persons, who observe these two rules relative to eating and drinking, cannot possibly be corrupted, and engender acute diseases, the sources of an untimely death, every man is bound to comply with them: for whoever acts otherwise, living a disorderly instead of a regular life, is constantly exposed to disease and mortality, as well in consequence of such disorders, as of others without number, each of which is capable of producing the same destructive effect.

It is, indeed, true, that even those, who observe the two rules relating to diet, the observance of which constitutes a sober life, may, by committing any one of the other irregularities, find himself the worse for it, for a day or two; but not so as to breed a fever. He may, likewise, be affected by the revolutions of the heavens; but neither the heavens, nor those irregularities, are capable of corrupting the humours of a temperate person; and it is but reasonable and natural it should be so, as the two irregularities of diet are interior, and the others exterior.

But as there are some persons, stricken in years, who are, notwithstanding, very gluttonous, and alledge that neither the quantity or quality of their diet makes any impression upon them, and therefore eat a great deal, and of every thing without distinction, and indulge themselves equally in point of drinking, because they do not know in what part of their bodies their stomachs are situated; such, no doubt, are beyond all measure sensual, and slaves to gluttony. To these I answer, that what they say is impossible in the nature of things, because it is impossible that every man, who comes into the world, should not bring with him a hot, a cold, or a temperate constitution; and that hot foods should agree with hot constitutions, cold with cold ones, and things that are not of a temperate nature, with temperate ones, is likewise impossible in nature. After all, these epicures must allow, that they are now and then out of order; and that they cure themselves by taking evacuating medicines and observing a strict diet. Whence it appears, that their being out of order is owing to their eating too much, and of things disagreeing with their stomachs.

There are other old gluttons, who say, that it is necessary they should eat and drink a great deal, to keep up their natural heat, which is constantly diminishing, as they advance in years; and that it is, therefore, necessary to eat heartily, and of such things as please their palate, be they hot, cold, or temperate; and that, were they to lead a sober life, it would be a short one. To these I answer, that our kind mother, nature, in order that old men may live still to a greater age, has contrived matters so, that they should be able to subsist on little, as I do; for, large quantities of food cannot be digested by old and feeble stomachs. Nor should such persons be afraid of shortening their days by eating too little, since when they happen to be indisposed, they recover by lessening the quantity of their food; for it is a trifle they eat, when confined to a regimen, by observing which they get rid of their disorder. Now, if by reducing themselves to a very small quantity of food, they recover from the jaws of death, how can they doubt but that with an increase of diet, still consistent however with sobriety, they will be able to support nature when in perfect health?

Others say, that it is better for a man to suffer every year three or four returns of his usual disorders, such as the gout, pain in the side, and the like, than be tormented the whole year by not indulging his appetite, and eating every thing his palate likes best; since, by a good regimen alone, he is sure to get the better of such attacks. To this I answer, that our natural heat growing less and less, as we advance in years, no regimen can retain virtue sufficient to conquer the malignity, with which disorders of repletion are ever attended; so that he must die, at last, of these periodical disorders, because they abridge life, as health prolongs it.

Others pretend, that it is much better to live ten years less, than not indulge one's appetite. To this I answer, that longevity ought to be highly valued by men of parts; as to others, it is no great matter if it is not duly prized by them, since they are a disgrace to mankind, so that their death is rather of service to the public. But it is a great misfortune, that men of bright parts should be cut off in that manner, since he, who is already a cardinal, might, perhaps, by living to eighty, attain the papal crown; and in the state, many, by living some years extraordinary, may acquire the ducal dignity; and so in regard to letters, by which a man may rise so as to be considered as a god upon earth; and the like in every other profession.

There are others, who, though their stomachs become weaker and weaker with respect to digestion, as they advance in years, cannot, however, be brought to retrench the quantity of their food, nay they rather increase it. And, because they find themselves unable to digest the great quantity of food, with which they must load their stomachs, by eating twice in the four and twenty hours, they make a resolution to eat but once, that the long interval between one meal and the other may enable them to eat at one sitting as much as they used to do in two: thus they eat till their stomachs, overburthened with much food, pall, and sicken, and change the superfluous food into bad humours, which kill a man before his time. I never knew any person, who led that kind of life, live to be very old. All these old men I have been speaking of would live long, if, as they advanced in years, they lessened the quantity of their food, and eat oftener, but little at a time; for old stomachs cannot digest large quantities of food; old men changing, in that respect, to children, who eat several times in the four and twenty hours.

Others say, that temperance may, indeed, keep a man in health, but that it cannot prolong his life. To this I answer, that experience proves the contrary; and that I myself am a living instance of it. It cannot be said, that sobriety is apt to shorten one's days, as sickness does; and that the latter abbreviates life, is most certain. Moreover, a constant succession of good health is preferable to frequent sickness, as the radical moisture is thereby preserved. Hence it may be fairly concluded, that holy sobriety is the true parent of health and longevity.

O thrice holy sobriety, so useful to man, by the services thou renderest him! thou prolongest his days, by which means he greatly improves his understanding, and by such improvement he avoids the bitter fruits of sensuality, which are an enemy to reason, man's peculiar privilege: those bitter fruits are the passions and perturbations of the mind. Thou, moreover, freest him from the dreadful thoughts of death. How greatly is thy faithful disciple indebted to thee, since by thy assistance he enjoys this beautiful expanse of the visible world, which is really beautiful to such as know how to view it with the philosophic eye, as thou has enabled me to do. Nor could I, at any other time of life, even when I was young, but altogether debauched by an irregular life, perceive its beauties, though I spared no pains or expence to enjoy every season of life. But I found that all the pleasures of that age had their alloy; so that I never knew, till I grew old, that the world was beautiful. O truly happy life, which, over and above all these favours conferred on thine old man, hast so improved and perfected his stomach, that he has now a better relish for his dry bread, than he had formerly and in his youth, for the most exquisite dainties: and all this he has compassed by acting rationally, knowing, that bread is, above all things, man's proper food, when seasoned by a good appetite; and, whilst a man leads a sober life, he may be sure of never wanting that natural sauce; because, by always eating little, the stomach, not being much burthened, need not wait long to have an appetite. It is for this reason, that dry bread relishes so well with me; and I know it from experience, and can with truth affirm, I find such sweetness in it, that I should be afraid of sinning against temperance, were it not for my being convinced of the absolute necessity of eating it, and that we cannot make use of a more natural food. And thou, kind parent Nature, who actest so lovingly by thy aged offspring, in order to prolong his days, hast contrived matters so in his favour, that he can live upon very little; and, in order to add to the favour, and do him still greater service, hast made him sensible, that, as in his youth he used to eat twice a day, when he arrived at old age, he ought to divide that food, of which he was accustomed before to make but two meals, into four; because, thus divided, it will be more easily digested; and, as in his youth he made but two meals in the day, he should, in his old age, make four, provided however he lessens the quantity, as his years increase. And this is what I do, agreeably to my own experience; and, therefore, my spirits, not oppressed by much food, but barely kept up, are always brisk; especially after eating, so that I am accustomed then to sing a song, and afterwards to write.

Nor do I ever find myself the worse for writing immediately after meals; nor is my understanding ever clearer; nor am I apt to be drowsy; the food I take being too small a quantity to send up any fumes to the brain. O, how advantageous it is to an old man to eat but little! Accordingly, I, who know it, eat but just enough to keep body and soul together; and the things I eat are as follow. First, bread, panado, some broth with an egg in it, or such other good kinds of soup or spoon-meat. Of flesh meat, I eat veal, kid, and mutton. I eat poultry of every kind. I eat partridges, and other birds, such as thrushes. I likewise eat fish; for instance, the goldney and the like, amongst sea fish; and the pike, and such like, amongst the fresh-water fish. All these things are fit for an old man; and, therefore, he ought to be content with them, and, considering their number and variety, not hanker after others. Such old men, as are too poor to allow themselves provisions of this kind, may do very well with bread, panado, and eggs; things, which no poor man can want, unless it be common beggars, and, as we call them, vagabonds, about whom we are not bound to make ourselves uneasy, since they have brought themselves to that pass by their indolence; and had better be dead than alive; for they are a disgrace to human nature. But, though a poor man should eat nothing but bread, panado, and eggs, there is no necessity for his eating more than his stomach can digest. And, whoever does not trespass in point of either quantity or quality, cannot die but by mere dissolution. O, what a difference there is between a regular and an irregular life! One gives longevity and health, the other produces diseases and untimely deaths.

O unhappy, wretched life, my sworn enemy, who art good for nothing but to murder those, who follow thee! How many of my dearest relations and friends hast thou robbed me of, in consequence of their not giving credit to me; relations and friends, whom I should now enjoy. But thou hast not been able to destroy me, according to thy wicked intent and purpose. I am still alive in spite of thee, and have attained to such an age, as to see around me eleven grandchildren, all of fine understanding, and amiable disposition; all given to learning and virtue; all beautiful in their persons and lovely in their manners; whom, had I obeyed thy dictates, I should never have beheld. Nor should I enjoy those beautiful and convenient apartments which I have built from the ground, with such a variety of gardens, as required no small time to attain their present degree of perfection. No! thy nature is to destroy those who follow thee, before they can see their houses or gardens so much as finished; whereas, I, to thy no small confusion, have already enjoyed mine for a great number of years. But, since thou art so pestilential a vice, as to poison and destroy the whole world; and I am determined to use my utmost endeavours to extirpate thee, at least in part; I have resolved to counteract thee so, that my eleven grandchildren shall take pattern after me; and thereby expose thee, for what thou really art, a most wicked, desperate, and mortal enemy of the children of men.

I, really, cannot help admiring, that men of fine parts, and such there are, who have attained a superior rank in letters or any other profession, should not betake themselves to a regular life, when they are arrived at the age of fifty or sixty; or as soon as they find themselves attacked by any of the foregoing disorders, of which they might easily recover; whereas, by being permitted to get a head, they become incurable. As to young men, I am no way surprised by them, since, the passions being strong at that age, they are of course the more easily overpowered by their baleful influence. But after fifty, our lives should, in every thing, be governed by reason, which teaches us, that the consequences of gratifying our palate and our appetite are disease and death. Were this pleasure of the palate lasting, it would be some excuse; but it is so momentary, that there is scarce any distinguishing between the beginning and the end of it; whereas the diseases it produces are very durable. But it must be a great contentment to a man of sober life, to be able to reflect that, in the manner he lives, he is sure, that what he eats, will keep him in good health, and be productive of no disease or infirmity.

Now I was willing to make this short addition to my treatise, founded on new reasons; few persons caring to peruse long-winded discourses; whereas short tracts have a chance of being read by many; and I wish that many may see this addition, to the end that its utility may be more extensive.

AN EARNEST EXHORTATION; WHEREIN The author uses the strongest arguments to persuade all men to embrace a regular and sober life, in order to attain old age, in which they may enjoy all the favours and blessings, that God, in his goodness, vouchsafes to bestow upon mortals.

Not to be wanting to my duty, that duty incumbent upon every man; and not to lose at the same time the satisfaction I feel in being useful to others, I have resolved to take up my pen, and inform those, who, for want of conversing with me, are strangers to what those know and see, with whom I have the pleasure of being acquainted. But, as certain things may appear, to some persons, scarce credible, nay impossible, though actually fact, I shall not fail to relate them for the benefit of the public. Wherefore, I say, being (God be praised) arrived at my ninety-fifth year, and still finding myself sound and hearty, content and chearful, I never cease thanking the Divine Majesty for so great a blessing; considering the usual fate of other old men. These scarce attain the age of seventy, without losing their health and spirits; growing melancholy and peevish; and continually haunted by the thoughts of death; apprehending their last hour from one day to another, so that it is impossible to drive such thoughts out of their mind; whereas such things give me not the least uneasiness; for, indeed, I cannot, at all, make them the object of my attention, as I shall hereafter more plainly relate. I shall, besides, demonstrate the certainty I have of living to an hundred. But, to render this dissertation more methodical, I shall begin by considering man at his birth; and from thence accompany him through every stage of life to his grave.

I, therefore, say, that some come into the world with the stamina of life so weak, that they live but a few days, or months, or years; and it cannot be clearly known, to what such shortness of life is owing; whether to some defect in the father or the mother, in begetting them; or to the revolutions of the heavens; or to the defect of nature, subject, as she is, to the celestial influence. For, I could never bring myself to believe, that nature, common parent of all, should be partial to any of her children. Therefore, as we cannot assign causes, we must be content with reasoning from the effects, such as they daily appear to our view.

Others are born sound, indeed, and full of spirits; but, notwithstanding, with a poor weakly constitution; and of these some live to the age of ten; others to twenty; others to thirty or forty; yet they do not live to extreme old age. Others, again, bring into the world a perfect constitution, and live to old age; but it is generally, as I have already said, an old age full of sickness and sorrow; for which they are to thank themselves; because they most unreasonably presume on the goodness of their constitution; and cannot by any means be brought to depart, when brought to depart, when grown old, from the mode of life they pursued in their younger days; as if they still retained all their primitive vigour. Nay, they intend to live as irregularly when past the meridian of life, as they did all the time of their youth; thinking they shall never grow old, nor their constitution ever be impaired. Neither do they consider, that their stomach has lost its natural heat; and that they should, on that account, pay a greater regard to the quality of what they eat, and what wines they drink; and likewise to the quantity of each, which they ought to lessen; whereas, on the contrary, they are for increasing it; saying, that, as we lose our health and vigour by growing old, we should endeavour to repair the loss by increasing the quantity of our food, since it is by sustenance that man is preserved.

In this, nevertheless, they are greatly mistaken, since, as the natural heat lessens as a man grows in years, he should diminish the quantity of his meat and drink; nature, especially at that period, being content with little. Nay, though they have all the reason to believe this to be the case, they are so obstinate as to think otherwise, and still follow their usual disorderly life. But were they to relinquish it in due time, and betake themselves to a regular and sober course, they would not grow infirm in their old age, but would continue, as I am, strong and hearty, considering how good and perfect a constitution it has pleased the Almighty to bestow upon them; and would live to the age of one hundred and twenty. This has been the case of others, who, as we read in many authors, have lived a sober life, and, of course, were born with this perfect constitution; and had it been my lot to enjoy such a constitution, I should make no doubt of attaining the same age. But, as I was born with feeble stamina, I am afraid I shall not outlive an hundred. Were others, too, who are also born with an infirm constitution, to betake themselves to a regular life, as I have done, they would attain the age of one hundred and upwards, as will be my case.

And this certainty of being able to live a great age is, in my opinion, a great advantage, and highly to be valued; none being sure to live even a single hour, except such as adhere to the rules of temperance. This security of life is built on good and true natural reasons, which can never fail; it being impossible in the nature of things, that he, who leads a sober and regular life, should breed any sickness, or die of an unnatural death, before the time, at which it is absolutely impossible he should live. But sooner he cannot die, as a sober life has the virtue to remove all the usual causes of sickness, and sickness cannot happen without a cause; which cause being removed, sickness is, likewise, removed; and sickness being removed, an untimely and violent death must be prevented.

And there is no doubt, that temperance has the virtue and efficacy to remove such causes; for since health and sickness, life and death, depend on the good or bad quality of the humours, temperance corrects their vicious tendencies, and renders them perfect, being possessed of the natural power of making them unite and hold together, so as to render them inseperable, and incapable of alteration and fermenting; circumstances, which engender cruel fevers, and end in death. It is true, indeed, and it would be a folly to deny it, that, let our humours be originally ever so good, time, which consumes every thing, cannot fail to consume and exhaust them; and that man, as soon as that happens, must die of a natural death; but yet without sickness, as will be my case, who shall die at my appointed time, when these humours shall be consumed, which they are not at present. Nay, they are still perfect; nor is it possible they should be otherwise in my present condition, when I find myself hearty and content, eating with a good appetite, and sleeping soundly. Moreover, all my faculties are as good as ever, and in the highest perfection; my understanding clearer and brighter than ever; my judgment sound; my memory tenacious; my spirits good; and my voice, the first thing which is apt to fail in others, grown so strong and sonorous, that I cannot help chanting out loud my prayers morning and night, instead of whispering and muttering them to myself, as was formerly my custom.

And these are all so many true and sure signs and tokens, that my humours are good, and cannot waste but with time, as all those, who converse with me, conclude. O, how glorious this life of mine is like to be, replete with all the felicities which man can enjoy on this side of the grave; and even exempt from that sensual brutality which age has enabled my better reason to banish; because where reason resides, there is no room for sensuality, nor for its bitter fruits, the passions, and perturbations of the mind, with a train of disagreeable apprehensions. Nor yet can the thoughts of death find room in my mind, as I have no sensuality to nourish such thoughts. Neither can the death of grandchildren and other relations and friends make any impression on me, but for a moment or two; and then it is over. Sill less am I liable to be cast down by losses in point of fortune (as many have seen to their no small surprise.) And this is a happiness not to be expected by any but such as attain old age by sobriety, and not in consequence of a strong constitution; and such may moreover expect to spend their days happily, as I do mine, in a perpetual round of amusement and pleasure. And how is it possible a man should not enjoy himself, who meets with no crosses or disappointments in his old age, such as youth is constantly plagued with, and from which, I shall presently shew, I have the happiness of being exempt?

The first of these is to do service to my country. O! what a glorious amusement, in which I find infinite delight, as I thereby shew her the means of improving her important estuary or harbour beyond the possibility of its filling for thousands of years to come; so as to secure to Venice her surprising and miraculous title of a maiden city, as she really is; and the only one in the whole world: she will, moreover, thereby, add to the lustre of her great and excellent surname of queen of the sea: such is my amusement; and nothing is wanting to make it complete. Another amusement of mine, is that of shewing this maid and queen, in what manner she may abound with provisions, by improving large tracts of land, as well marshes, as barren sands, to great profit. A third amusement, and an amusement too, without any alloy, is the shewing how Venice, though already so strong as to be in a manner impregnable, may be rendered still stronger; and, though extremely beautiful, may still increase in beauty; though rich, may acquire more wealth, and may be made to enjoy better air, though her air is excellent. These three amusements, all arising from the idea of public utility, I enjoy in the highest degree. And who can say, that they admit of any alloy, as in fact they do not? Another comfort I enjoy, is, that having lost a considerable part of my income, of which my grandchildren had been unfortunately robbed, I by mere dint of thought, which never sleeps, and without any fatigue of body, and very little of mind, have found a true and infallable method of repairing such loss more than double, by the means of that most commendable of arts, agriculture. Another comfort I still enjoy is to think, that my treatise on temperance, which I wrote in order to be useful to others, is really so, as many assure me by word of mouth, mentioning that it has proved extremely useful to them, as it in fact appears to have been, whilst others inform me by letter, that, under God, they are indebted to me for life. Still another comfort I enjoy, is that of being able to write with my own hand; for, I write enough to be of service to others, both on architecture, and agriculture. I, likewise, enjoy another satisfaction, which is that of conversing with men of bright parts and superior understanding, from whom, even at this advanced period of life, I learn something. What a comfort is this, that, old as I am, I should be able, without the least fatigue, to study the most important, sublime, and difficult subjects!

I must farther add, though it may appear impossible to some, and may be so in some measure, that at this age I enjoy, at once, two lives; one terrestrial, which I possess in fact; the other celestial, which I possess in thought; and this thought is equal to actual enjoyment, when founded upon things we are sure to attain, as I ams sure to attain that celestial life, through the infinite goodness and mercy of God. Thus, I enjoy this terrestrial life, in consequence of my sobriety and temperance, virtues so agreeable to the Deity; and I enjoy, by the grace of the same Divine Majesty, the celestial, which he makes me anticipate in thought; a thought so lovely, as to fix me entirely on this object, the enjoyment of which I hold and affirm to be of the utmost certainty. And I hold that dying, in the manner I expect, is not really death, but a passage of the soul from this earthly life to a celestial, immortal, and infinitely perfect existence. Neither can it be otherwise: and this thought is so superlatively sublime, that it can no longer stoop to low and worldly objects, such as the death of this body, being intirely taken up with the happiness of living a celestial and divine life; whence it is, that I enjoy two lives. Nor can the terminating of so high a gratification, which I enjoy in this life, give me any concern; it rather affords me infinite pleasure, as it will be only to make room for another, glorious and immortal life.

Now, it is possible, that any one should grow tired of so great a comfort and blessing, as this which I really enjoy; and which every on else might enjoy by leading the life I have led? an example which every one has it in his power to follow; for I am but a mere man, and no saint; a servant of God, to whom so regular a life is extremely agreeable.

And, whereas many embrace a spiritual and contemplative life, which is holy and commendable, the chief employment of those who lead it being to celebrate the praises of God; O, that the would likewise, betake themselves intirely to a regular and sober life! how much more agreeable would they render themselves in the sight of God! What a much greater honour and ornament would the be to the world! They would then be considered as saints, indeed, upon earth, as those primitive Christians were led, who joined sobriety to so recluse a life. By living, like them, to the age of one hundred and twenty, they might, like them, expect, by the power of God, to work numberless miracles; and they would, besides, enjoy constant health and spirits, and be always happy within themselves; whereas they are now, for the most part, infirm, melancholy, and dissatisfied. Now, as some of these people think, that these are trials sent them by God Almighty, with a view of promoting their salvation, that they may do penance, in this life, for their past errors, I cannot help saying, that, in my opinion, they are greatly mistaken. For I can by no means believe, that it is agreeable to the Deity, that man, his favourite creature, should live infirm, melancholy, and dissatisfied, but rather enjoy good health and spirits, and be always content within himself. In this manner did the holy fathers live, and by such conduct did they daily render themselves more acceptable to the Divine Majesty, so as to work the great and surprising miracles we read in history. How beautiful, how glorious a scene should we then behold! far more beautiful than in those antient times, because we now abound with so many religious orders and monasteries, which did not then exist; and were the members of these communities to lead a temperate life, we should then behold such a number of venerable old men, as would create surprise. Nor would they trespass against their rules; they would rather improve upon them; since every religious community allows its subjects bread, wine, and sometimes eggs (some of them allow meat) besides soups made with vegetables, sallets, fruit, and cakes, things which often disagree with them, and even shorten their lives. But, as they are allowed such things by their rules, they freely make use of them; thinking, perhaps, that it would be wrong to abstain from them, whereas it would not. It would rather be commendable, if, after the age of thirty, they abstained from such food, confined themselves to bread, wine, broths and eggs: for this is the true method of preserving men of a bad constitution; and it is a life of more indulgence than that led by the holy fathers of the desert, who subsisted intirely on wild fruits and roots, and drank nothing but pure water; and, nevertheless, lived, as I have already mentioned, in good health and spirits, and always happy within themselves. Were those of our days to do the same, they would, like them, find the road to heaven much easier; for it is always open to every faithful Christian, as our Saviour Jesus Christ left it, when he came down upon earth to shed his precious blood, in order to deliver us from the tyrannical servitude of the devil; and all through his immense goodness.

So that, to make an end of this discourse, I say, that since length of days abounds with so many favours and blessings, and I happen to be one of those who are arrived at that state, I cannot (as I would not willingly want charity) but give testimony in favour of it, and solemnly assure all mankind, that I really enjoy a great deal more than what I now mention; and that I have no other reason for writing, but that of demonstrating the great advantages which arise from longevity, to the end that their own conviction may induce them to observe those excellent rules of temperance and sobriety. And therefore I never cease to raise my voice, crying out to you, my friends: may your days be long, that you may be the better servants to the Almighty!

LETTER FROM SIGNOR LEWIS CORNARO, TO THE RIGHT REVEREND BARBARO, PATRIARCH ELECT OF AQUILEIA.

The human understanding must certainly have something of the divine in its constitution and frame. How divine the invention of conversing with an absent friend by the help of writing! How divinely it is contrived by nature, that men, though at a great distance, should see one another with the intellectual eye, as I now see your lordship! By means of this contrivance, I shall endeavour to entertain you with with matters of the greatest moment.

It is true, that I shall speak of nothing but what I have already mentioned; but it was not at the age of ninety-one, to which I have now attained; a thing I cannot help taking notice of, because as I advance in years, the sounder and heartier I grow, to the amazement of all the world. I, who can account for it, am bound to shew, that a many may enjoy a terrestrial paradise after eighty; which I enjoy; but it is not to be obtained except by temperance and sobriety, virtues so acceptable to the Almighty, because they are enemies to sensuality, and friends to reason.

Now, my lord, to begin, I must tell you, that, within these few days past, I have been visited by many of the learned doctors of this university, as well physicians and philosophers, who were well acquainted with my age, my life, and manners; knowing how stout, hearty, and gay I was; and in what perfection all my faculties still continued; likewise my memory, spirits, and understanding; and even my voice and teeth. They knew, besides, that I constantly employed eight hours every day in writing treatises, with my own hand, on subjects useful to mankind, and spent many hours in walking and singing. O, my lord, how melodious my voice is grown! were you to hear me chant my prayers; and that to my lyre, after the example of David, I am certain it would give you great pleasure, my voice is so musical. Now, when they told me that they had been already acquainted with all these particulars, they added, that it was, indeed, next to a miracle, how I could write so much, and upon subjects that required both judgement and spirit. And, indeed, my lord, it is incredible, what satisfaction and pleasure I have in these compositions. But, as I write to be useful, your lordship may easily conceive what pleasure I enjoy. They concluded by telling me, that I ought not to be looked upon as a person advanced in years, since all my occupations were those of a young man; and, by no means, like those of other aged persons, who, when they have reached eighty, are reckoned decrepid. Such, moreover, are subject, some to the gout, some to the sciatica, and some to other complaints, to be relieved from which they must undergo such a number of painful operations, as cannot but render life extremely disagreeable. And, if, by chance, one of them happens to escape a long illness, his faculties are impaired, and he cannot see or hear so well; or else fails in some or other of the corporeal faculties, he cannot walk, or his hands shake; and, supposing him exempt from these bodily infirmities, his memory, his spirits, or his understanding fail him; he is not chearful, pleasant, and happy within himself, as I am.

Besides all these blessings, I mentioned another, which I enjoyed; and so great a blessing, that they were all amazed at it, since it is altogether beside the usual course of nature. This blessing is, that I had already lived fifty years, in spite of a most powerful and mortal enemy, which I can by no means conquer, because it is natural, or an occult quality implanted in my body by nature; and this is, that every year, from the beginning of July till the end of August, I cannot drink any wine of whatever kind or country; for, besides being during these two months quite disgustful to my palate, it disagrees with my stomach. Thus losing my milk, for wine is, indeed, the milk of old age; and having nothing to drink, for no change or preparation of waters can have the virtue of wine, nor of course do me any good; having nothing, I say, to drink, and my stomach being therefore disordered, I can eat but very little; and this spare diet, with the want of wine, reduces me, by the middle of August, extremely low; nor is the strongest capon broth, or any other remedy, of service to me; so that I am ready, through mere weakness, to sink into the grave. Hence they inferred, that were not the new wine, for I always take care to have some ready by the beginning of September, to come in so soon, I should be a dead man. But what surprized them still more was, that this new wine should have power sufficient to restore me, in two or three days, to that degree of health and strength, of which the old wine had robbed me; a fact, they themselves have been eye-witnesses of, within these few days; and which a man must see to believe it; insomuch that they could not help crying out; "Many of us, who are physicians, have visited him annually for several years past; and ten years ago, judged it impossible for him to live a year or two longer, considering what a mortal enemy he carried about him, and his advanced age; yet we do not find him so weak at present as he used to be." This singularity, and the many other blessings they see me enjoy, obliged them to confess, that the joining of such a number of favours was, with regard to me, a special grace conferred on me, at my birth, by nature, or by the stars; and to prove this to be a good conclusion, which it really is not (because not grounded on strong and sufficient reasons, but merely on their own opinions) they found themselves under a necessity to display their eloquence, and to say a great many fine things. Certain it is, my lord, that eloquence, in men of bright parts, has great power; so great, as to induce people to believe things which have neither actual nor possible existence. I had, however, great pleasure and satisfaction in hearing them; for, it must, no doubt, be a high entertainment to hear such men talk in that manner.

Another satisfaction, without the least mixture of alloy, I at the same time enjoyed, was to think, that age and experience are sufficient to make a man learned, who without them would know nothing; nor is it surprizing they should, since length of days is the foundation of true knowledge. Accordingly, it was by means of it alone I discovered their conclusion to be false. Thus, you see, my lord, how apt men are to deceive themselves in their judgement of things, when such judgement is not built upon a solid foundation. And, therefore, to undeceive them, and set them right, I made answer, that their conclusion was false, as I should actually convince them by proving, that the happiness I enjoyed was not confined to me, but common to all mankind, and that every man might equally enjoy it; since I was but a mere mortal, composed, like all others, of the four elements; and endued, besides existence and life, with rational and intellectual faculties, which are common to all men. For it has pleased the Almighty to bestow on his favourite creature man these extraordinary blessings and favours above other animals, which enjoy only the sensible perceptions; in order such blessings and favours my be the means of keeping him long in good health; so that length of days is a universal favour granted by the Deity, and not by nature and the stars.

But man being in his youthful days more of the sensual, than of the rational animal, is apt to yield to sensual impressions; and, when he afterwards arrives at the age of forty or fifty, he ought to consider, that he has attained the noon of life, by the vigour of his youth, and a good tone of stomach; natural blessings, which favoured him in ascending the hill; but that he must now think of going down, and approaching the grave, with a heavy weight of years on his back; and that old age is the reverse of youth, as much as order is the reverse of disorder. Hence it is requisite he should alter his mode of life in regard to the articles of eating and drinking, on which health and longevity depend. And as the first part of his life was sensual and irregular, the second should be the reverse; since nothing can subsist without order, especially the life of man, irregularity being without all doubt prejudicial, and regularity advantageous to the human species.

Besides, it is impossible in the nature of things, that the man, who is bent on indulging his palate and his appetite, should not be guilty of irregularity. Hence it was that to avoid this vice, as soon as I found myself arrived at maturer years, I embraced a regular and sober life. It is, no doubt, true, that I found some difficulty in compassing it; but, in order to conquer this difficulty, I beseeched the Almighty to grant me the virtue of sobriety; well knowing, that he would graciously hear my prayer. Then, considering, that when a man is about to undertake any thing of importance, which he knows he can compass, though not without difficulty, he may make it much easier to himself by being steady in his purpose; I pursued the same course. I endeavoured gradually to relinquish a disorderly life, and to accustom myself insensibly to the rules of temperance: and thus it came to pass that a sober and regular life no longer proved uneasy or disagreeable; though, on account of the weakness of my constitution, I tied myself down to such strict rules in regard to the quantity and quality of what I eat and drink.

But others, who happen to be blessed with a stronger temperament, may eat many other kinds of food, and in greater quantities; and so of wines; whereas, though their lives may still be sober, they will not be so confined as mine, but much more free. Now, on hearing these arguments, and examining the reasons on which they were founded, they all agreed that I had advanced nothing but what was true. Indeed the youngest of them said, that though he could not but allow the favour of advantages, I had been speaking of, to be common to all mankind, yet I enjoyed the special grace of being able to relinquish with ease one kind of life, and embrace another; a think which he knew by experience to be feasible; but as difficult to him as it had proved easy to me.

To this I replied, that, being a mortal like himself, I likewise found it a difficult task; but it did not become a person to shrink from a glorious but practicable undertaking, on account of the difficulties attending it, because in proportion to these difficulties, is the honour he acquires by it in the eye of man, and the merit in the sight of God. Our beneficent Creator is desirous, that, as he originally favoured human nature with longevity, we should all enjoy full advantage of his intentions; knowing, that, when a man has passed eighty, he is intirely exempt from the bitter fruits of sensual enjoyments, and is intirely governed by the dictates of reason. Vice and immorality must then leave him; hence God is willing he should live to a full maturity of years; and has ordained that whoever reaches his natural term, should end his days without sickness by mere dissolution, the natural way of quitting this mortal life to enter upon immortality, as will be my case. For I am sure to die chanting my prayers; nor do the dreadful thoughts of death give me the least uneasiness, though, considering my great age, it cannot be far distant, knowing, as I do, that I was born to die, and reflecting that such numbers have departed my life without reaching my age.

Nor does that other thought, inseperable from the former, namely the fear of those torments, to which wicked men are hereafter liable, give me any uneasiness; because I am a good Christian, and bound to believe, that I shall be saved by the virtue of the most sacred blood of Christ, which he has vouchsafed to shed, in order to free us from those torments. How beautiful is the life I lead! how happy my end! To this, the young gentleman, my antagonist, had nothing to reply, but that he was resolved to embrace a sober life, in order to follow my example; and that he had taken another, more important, resolution, which was, that, as he had been always very desirous to live to be old, so he was now equally impatient to reach that period, the sooner to enjoy the felicity of old age.

The great desire I had, my lord, to converse with you at this distance, has forced me to be prolix, and still obliges me to proceed; though not much farther. There are many sensualists, my lord, who say, that I have thrown away my time and trouble in writing a treatise on Temperance, and other discourses on the same subject, to induce men to lead a regular life; alledging, that it is impossible to conform to it, so that my treatise must answer as little purpose as that of Plato on government, who took a great deal of pains to recommend a thing impracticable; whence they inferred, that as his treatise was of no use, mine will share the same fate. Now this surprises me the more, as they may see by my treatise, that I had led a sober life for many years before I had composed it; and that I should never have composed it, had I not previously been convinced, that it was such a life as a man might lead; and being a virtuous life, would be of great service to him; so that I thought myself under an obligation to represent it in a true light. I have the satisfaction now to hear, that numbers, on seeing my treatise, have embraced such a life; and I have read, that many, in times past, have actually led it; so that the objection, to which Plato's treatise on government is liable, can be of no force against mine. But such sensualists, enemies to reason, and slaves to their passions, ought to think themselves well off, if, whilst they study to indulge their palate and their appetite, they do not contract long and painful diseases, and are not, many of them, overtaken by an untimely death.

FINIS

www.ingramcontent.com/pod-product-compliance
Lightning Source LLC
Chambersburg PA
CBHW071013290526
45795CB00005B/1791